The New Menu That Began My Mother's Recovery from COPD & Emphysema

Contents

Preface

First of all let me say I had no intention of writing this book. My intention was first get my mother well and then return to work in the software industry. I had started years earlier in an engineering position which eventually led me to the Information Technology industry, specifically focusing on sales and marketing of software.

When my mother was diagnosed with COPD I immediately began researching the disease online each evening. Sometimes I would only spend an hour and other times I would spend 6 or 8 hours.

One thing I noticed after only a month or so of researching was that I always ended up on medical and pharmaceutical controlled web sites. Once arriving there I soon found the same information I had read many times before. The disease is *"progressive"* yet they tell you there are ways of treating it. *"Progressive"* is apparently the new, politically correct term replacing *"terminal."*

They do not tell you that using these methods of treatment will not stop the disease progression. In some cases I did find web sites stating that it had been shown in clinical trials that a particular drug *"slowed the progress of the disease."* Not one web site claimed that the medications would stop the progress of the disease so, of course, there were also none claiming they would cure the disease.

At this point I realized we had a real problem. Most of these sites tell you that the disease is *"progressive"* and imply that this progression cannot be stopped. They also state that it is not known why COPD continues progressing even after the patient quits smoking.

Eventually my research began revealing information that I thought might help my mother. I call what I was doing *"research"* throughout the book when, in fact, it was data mining and curation. I find the information published by or about prominent researchers and their findings and then, where applicable, apply it to COPD. I did this since I was finding very little in the way of alternative research on COPD.

I found researchers like Fred Pescatore, M.D. a New York City physician who wrote the book, *"The Allergy and Asthma Cure."* On his patients' behalf, Dr. Pescatore had gone against medical protocols for treating these illnesses while his colleagues continued prescribing medications that do not provide a cure for these ailments.

Dr. Pescatore shows clearly that medications are not necessary or effective in treating asthma or allergies, long term. His 8-step cure restores the body to optimal health levels, restores the immune system and intestinal flora and eliminates both allergies and asthma in the end.

Once I found Dr. Pescatore I realized maybe it was possible there was a cure for COPD out there somewhere. I thought since Dr. Pescatore had developed a cure for allergies and asthma which was being ignored by the vast majority of doctors who still prescribed medications to their patients with these ailments.

I also realized that some of the natural treatments Dr. Pescatore used in his 8-step cure restored the body to optimal health. It seemed to me that this restoration to optimal health would be a good idea for anyone not just those suffering from some illness. I especially thought it would help my mother's condition.

I also found reassurance and hope with information published by a prominent researcher at Mayo Clinic, Hirohito Kita, M.D. Dr. Kita published his findings in 1999 stating that 96% of sinusitis (the inflammation of the sinuses) is caused by a fungal infection.

Sinusitis is a common problem associated with supplemental oxygen use provided by an oxygen concentrator machine. The problem arises with the continued use of the same breathing tube which becomes infected with fungi and/or mold over time. Changing these breathing tubes every week will eliminate this recurring sinusitis problem.

Out of desperation when my mother was at her worst, I adopted a diet laid out by Dr. Pescatore and Dr. Kenneth Hunter, a Microbiologist and cancer researcher at the University of Nevada School of Medicine. Both of these researchers were adamant about the need for eliminating sugar from the diet along with those foods that convert to sugar in only a few biochemical steps.

This diet began my mother's recovery from COPD. These researchers had ignored the established, ineffective medical treatments for the diseases they were treating and found amazing success with alternative treatments that provided healing and cures for their patients. Applying much of this research to COPD provided additional improvements for my mother and to-date, many thousands of others who were suffering from this debilitating illness.

I praise God for leading me to these researchers and this information. Without Him I do not believe this book or my mother's recovery would have been possible. You see, I compiled over 30,000 pages of information in my 4 and a half years of research. My mother was already in End Stage Emphysema and I knew she did not have much time left. I asked God to lead me to some information that would help my mother. What I am saying is that the book, *"How I Reversed My Mom's Emphysema"* is the result of His grace not my research.

Introduction

When my mother was diagnosed with COPD I was very concerned. I knew the disease was terminal or *"progressive"* as they call it now. As I began researching the disease I also observed my mother carefully as her condition deteriorated.

Knowing she was not smoking cigarettes any more I could not understand why the disease was progressing. After asking the doctors I realized they did not know why the disease was progressing either. They said the disease progression of COPD was a mystery. They would follow this statement with something about slowing the progress of the disease with prescription medications.

I wanted a way of stopping the disease from progressing not just slowing it down! I wasn't interested in prolonging my mother's suffering if she would die from the disease anyway. I noticed that over many months the amount of supplemental oxygen she required increased meaning the disease had progressed further. I noticed along with the increased supplemental oxygen requirement her meal size decreased resulting in weight loss.

It seemed like something was growing or proliferating in her lungs and none of the medications were stopping it. My mother's doctors were not even addressing this possibility yet they felt comfortable embracing this *"big mystery"* scenario. After all, it sold lots of drugs and they made lots of money. I was not comfortable with this complete failure of the medical industry and instead put all my attention into solving this big mystery!

After obtaining a copy of her medical record I saw that her weight had either stayed the same or dropped a pound or two on each successive visit to her doctor over the previous two years. In addition, I could see that the weight loss was accelerating.

What if this disease was nothing more than some pathogen proliferating in the lungs, which if stopped, would halt the progression of this disease?

This sounded more logical than the *"big mystery"* explanation the medical and pharmaceutical industries were basing their treatments on. You will read in the following chapters how I expanded this idea into a hypothesis and then into a "disease progression model" which, I believe, explains not only how the disease progresses but also how it can be stopped.

If you were hoping for a magic bullet or miracle drug that would eliminate this disease overnight without any real personal involvement, you will be disappointed with this book. However, if you take the realistic approach and realize that the situation you are in with this disease is a result of everything you have done in your life up to this point.

Hopefully, you also realize that beating this disease will require a drastic change in lifestyle. Once I realized this fact with regards to my mother, I realized it would take global changes in her lifestyle not just putting the cigarettes down.

Chapter 1: My Hypothesis

When I thought logically about what I was observing it occurred to me that maybe smoking introduced this unknown pathogen into the lungs that began proliferating upon its arrival and continued proliferating even if the patient quit smoking.

This would explain why my mother's emphysema and COPD continued progressing even though she had quit smoking. I reasoned that as this unknown pathogen proliferated, her body adapted by distending her lungs creating additional surface area for gas exchange (breathing). This proliferation of the pathogen followed by further distention of her lungs could have been going on for years, even decades before causing these serious and detectable problems.

The distending lungs would explain the "barrel chest" condition common with emphysema and COPD patients. My mother's distending lungs eventually began crowding her stomach little by little, causing the decrease in her meal size and her subsequent weight loss.

This was making so much more sense than what the doctors were telling me and what the pharmaceutical industry was claiming. I felt like the research was finally revealing some helpful information and I now had a logical "cause of disease" model that I could pursue with this newly established hypothesis. I already knew I could not rely on medications developed for treating the "effects" of this disease. Attacking the "cause" of COPD was my only hope of helping my mother survive this disease.

I remember the words of Arthur Schopenhauer (1788 – 1860), a German philosopher known for his philosophical clarity. I believe he made one of the most valuable observations on the shifting of human views on truth as he stated that all truth goes through three steps:

1.   First, it is ridiculed.
2.   Second, it is violently opposed.
3.   Finally, it is accepted as self-evident

I think we are somewhere between number 1 and number 2 right now. Hopefully we will arrive at number 3 very soon!

Chapter 2: The New Menu

After I read Dr. Hunter's research and other articles stating that cancer is a pathogen and pathogens eat sugar, I started thinking about this. If there was some unknown pathogen proliferating in my mother's lungs, the sugar in her diet might be feeding it.

Also, according to both Dr. Hunter and Dr. Pescatore, eliminating sugar along with grains and simple carbohydrates was necessary because foods made from grains like bread, cereal and pasta along with simple carbohydrates, are metabolized into sugar in only a few biochemical steps.

Starving the pathogen that I believed was causing the progression of my mother's emphysema and COPD would require eliminating all of these foods from her diet.

At this stage I was desperate. I had made sure my mother took all the prescribed medications and did all the required nebulizer treatments for the previous two years and yet I watched as she deteriorated down to *"End Stage Emphysema."*

Even though changing my mother's diet to this very restrictive one made logical sense, I truly did not think it would make much of a difference at this late stage. Maybe by this time in my mother's illness I had been swayed by the doctors' insistence that diet and supplements would not and could not cause any appreciable improvements in my mother's condition even though Harvard Medical School said they could.

I switched both of us to this New Menu anyway. I could not just sit back and watch her die. I knew I must do something and I realized the food on the New Menu was all healthy and therefore, could not hurt her.

We already had a lot of bread, cereal, potatoes, and pasta in the house so instead of throwing it out and wasting food I included it into our meals less and less until we had exhausted our supply. This was our 10 day transition period.

After these foods were gone I no longer bought them. I did not tell my mother we were on a special diet because I knew she would complain. Instead I made meals without the foods we were eliminating and did not bring up the fact that we were not having bread or potatoes or toast or some other eliminated food.

The Improvements Begin

After our 10 day transition, we were on the New Menu full time. The amazing thing was that after only two more weeks I began seeing improvements in my mother's condition! These improvements were subtle but they were noticeable and they were permanent!

She was still on 4 liters of supplemental oxygen however, she no longer gasped for air after walking from her bedroom into the kitchen. Her mood had improved and she was eating and sleeping a little more than she was two weeks earlier.

"The real significance of these improvements was that they were the first improvements my mother had shown since her diagnosis!"

In the early stages of emphysema my mother's deterioration was slow enough that I could not tell from day to day whether the medications and treatments prescribed by her doctors were improving her condition or not. I mistakenly assumed they were providing slow, steady improvement in her condition.

After reading information published by the drug manufacturers I realized their only claim was that the medications would *"slow the progress"* of the disease. They made no claims that these medications and treatments would *"stop"* or *"cure"* the disease.

It amazed me how many of these COPD patients thought they were getting better by taking these medications and performing the regular nebulizer treatments.

Once I learned the drugs were not curing the disease or even stopping its progress, I was very disappointed. I started thinking maybe my hypothesis was correct. Maybe there was some unknown pathogen proliferating in my mother's lungs and this New Menu was slowly taking away its food supply. Maybe we were reversing this disease process even though the doctors had said doing so was impossible.

More than $1200 in medications and treatments every month for more than 2 years had provided nothing more than temporary relief from symptoms. Now the first subtle signs of actual improvement were materializing and they were a result of a change in diet! Granted, the diet change was a drastic one. Still the improvements I was seeing in my mother's condition surprised me.

I couldn't believe the medical industry had not even thought of trying this change in diet! Maybe it centered on the fact that no company or organization would provide the funding for a study showing how diet could begin reversing emphysema and COPD. I guess since there was no profit in gathering this information, no one had bothered.

Main Course: Healthy Meats and Fish

Our main course consisted of healthy, uncontaminated protein such as beef, pork, chicken and fish. Some people eat lamb and goat meat which is fine if you like these meats. Personally, I no longer eat pork however, my mother had grown up on it and she enjoyed it so I included it in our meals occasionally.

By *"uncontaminated"* I mean animals that have not been given antibiotics or steroids. Most protein sources available at the local grocery stores are full of antibiotics and steroids. This includes the beef, pork and chicken.

More recently, fish have been raised in fish farms instead of being caught in the wild. Fish from fish farms are most likely fed antibiotics and steroids along with cost-effective food that may or may not be healthy.

Generally, fish farms have 8 to 10 times the number of fish in a given volume of water than what is found in the wild. This is done for the purpose of increasing production and profits, not because it produces healthier food for us. In fact, it has been shown that the nutrients are greatly reduced in farm raised fish! For this reason I avoid all fish that are *"farm raised."*

Finding protein sources that do not contain antibiotics and steroids can present a challenge and once you find them paying for them can create an even bigger challenge. If cows, pigs and chickens are not fed steroids they do not weigh near as much when butchered making the cost per pound of the meat much higher.

These animals are generally fed antibiotics because they put 4 or 5 times the number of animals in any given area than what you might find at an organic farm. If one of the animals gets an infection or an illness, the antibiotics kill the bacteria and prevent the infection from spreading to all the other animals. At least that is the theory. The way these animals are raised is very cruel. They have such a small area they can barely move.

If you want a healthier choice see if the grocery stores in your area offer a higher grade of meats that have not been given antibiotics or steroids. These meats are probably not the absolute highest quality but they are better than what you normally find at grocery stores.

The highest grade meats will include words and phrases like *"grass fed," "grass finished"* and *"free range."* All of these terms will generally mean a higher price and also a much higher grade of meat. Your local health foods store is a good place for these higher quality, higher priced meats.

Once I realized this I stopped buying regular meats and stuck with the antibiotic-free and steroid-free meats. While I did not notice any improvements that I could specifically attribute to these healthier protein sources, I knew they were instrumental in continuing my mother's improvement and recovery.

Even meats that say they were grass fed are not generally *"grass finished."* What this means is that these animals were fed corn during the six weeks prior to butchering.

I always thought finishing with corn was fine until I read an article in the Journal of the American Medical Association (JAMA) written by Ruth Edsell, M.D. Dr. Edsell stated that corn is universally contaminated with *Aspergillus* mold. She said that *Aspergillus* mold produces *aflatoxin B1*, one of the most carcinogenic substances known to man. It is known to cause colon cancer and should be avoided at all costs.

When the corn is taken out of the grain elevator it is sprayed with steam which kills the *Aspergillus* mold but not the *aflatoxin B1* it has produced. This means that any animal that is *"finished"* with corn is consuming this *aflatoxin B1*.

I was very careful in choosing these protein sources after reading the truth about them. It seems that food companies don't mind compromising quality and our health if it means more profits for them and their investors.

I typically fried fish or chicken once a week or so. With my mom sick I needed an alternate method of preparing these meats that was tasty and healthy. The solution I found was using marinade.

I began buying dry packets of marinade at the local discount grocery along with olive oil and balsamic vinegar. I used either balsamic vinegar or apple cider vinegar. I found out recently that olive oil breaks down when heated and it would have been healthier if I had used coconut oil because of its higher flash point. Coconut oil will break down also but at much higher temperatures than olive oil.

I am not sure that olive oil breaks down when baking at 350 degrees Fahrenheit. I think the problem occurs with much hotter temperatures like when stir frying. I prepared stir fry once a week using the softer vegetables including yellow squash, zucchini squash and white onions and either marinated beef or chicken or I used green, red, yellow and orange peppers with white onions and the marinated beef or chicken.

When stir frying I found it worked better if I used vegetables that had about the same consistency and required approximately the same cooking time so my mother did not have trouble chewing any of them. I found out recently that zucchini squash and yellow squash are both commonly genetically modified (GMO). Now that I know that, I no longer use them.

The meats, or protein sources, I generally marinated and then baked or grilled. As I mentioned, once a week or so I would prepare stir fry. I also used the crock pot on occasion since it was very easy and filled the house with the smell of the seasoning all day while it was cooking.

What We Drank

Deciding what we should drink would have been more difficult since so many prepared drinks contain sugar, high fructose corn syrup or artificial sweeteners except my mother doesn't drink much other than coffee, water and milk. My personal opinion, and the opinion of many other health advocates, is that artificial sweeteners are not a viable alternative to sugar cravings. Studies show that these sweeteners actually increase sugar cravings.

We stayed primarily with water, milk in moderation and coffee which my mother must have every morning or she quickly changes from a 100 pound elderly woman into an 800 pound gorilla.

Even though the coffee was very acidic, in general, I gave it to her anyway. I already knew I must pick my battles carefully. My mother does not like her coffee with sugar so that was not an issue.

I have now been drinking my coffee every morning without sugar for about 10 years and I still hate every cup. I drink it without sugar anyway. I did not have COPD but I knew that eating sugar would compromise my health whether I was sick with a debilitating illness or not.

As I mentioned, my mother does not like much liquid with her meal so it was not difficult eliminating sugary drinks. Admittedly, this was probably the only easy step in the whole process of getting my mother well and keeping her on the New Menu.

Side Dishes – Fresh Vegetables

Along with the marinated, baked or grilled meats I always had a vegetable or two that I steamed. Sometimes I would steam carrots and green beans together in the steamer and sometimes I just prepared one vegetable.

I always started with a fresh vegetable and steamed it. I never used canned vegetables since there is virtually no nutritional value left once the canning process is completed. The exception to this rule is vegetables that you can at home and purposely prepare in a healthy way.

Occasionally I would use frozen vegetables which are a good second choice if fresh vegetables are unavailable. I would visit the local vegetable market and the farmer's market every week, sometimes twice in the same week, making sure we always had a stock of fresh vegetables for steaming, for stir fry and for salads.

I divided the fresh vegetables in half. One half went into salads and the other half I steamed. My mother had problems with her teeth so the hard vegetables like broccoli and carrots I steamed whereas the zucchini and yellow squash were much softer so I cut them up for salads.

I bought one large bowl and lined it with paper towels. In it I put prepared Romaine lettuce. I used Romaine lettuce because 3 leaves of Romaine lettuce contain 100% of the vitamin B complex that our bodies need for the entire day. Since vitamin B complex is water-soluble I gave my mother two of these Romaine lettuce salads each day, one at lunch and one at dinner. Some people think that supplementing with a B complex vitamin is the same as eating these Romaine salads.

What I found in researching vitamin B was that most vitamin tablets include *"folic acid"* which is made in a lab and it is *"folate"* that occurs in nature. I remember reading a book by Dr. Reuben many years ago entitled, *"Everything You Always Wanted to Know About Nutrition."* In the book Dr. Reuben stated that you may not think your body knows the difference between these laboratory chemicals and their natural counterparts, but it does.

I cut up the vegetables and put them each in separate container lined with paper towels. With this arrangement, once I had all the vegetables cut up and in their respective containers, I could make a fresh salad in a matter of a minute or two. If one of the vegetables went bad I would throw it out and retain the others.

In the beginning I made up the entire salad with all the cut up vegetables mixed together but I soon noticed that after two days it looked much less appetizing. By keeping all the vegetables separate the salads looked freshly made every time. By preparing the vegetables in this way my mother could have a custom made salad each time she ate one. Maybe she did not want red peppers in her salad this time so I could simply leave them out.

If you have turned on the television and caught any news programs over the last few years you have probably seen the acronym GMO. GMO stands for "Genetically Modified Organism" and there are mixed opinions as to whether they are healthy or not. My personal opinion is that they are not. The EU (European Union) will not allow GMO foods in their jurisdiction. They do not recognize them as safe for human consumption. I don't believe they even allow them as animal feed.

Of course, the United States allows these products both for human and animal consumption. I prefer going to the local Farmer's Market for produce. There is also an Organic Farmer's Market close by so I have a few choices for healthy vegetables. If you do not have these choices available, check your local health foods store for these healthy vegetables.

Even if they do not sell them they can probably recommend places where you can find them. Fresh, uncooked vegetables contain enzymes that are extremely beneficial to everyone, especially someone with a debilitating illness like COPD and emphysema. Cooking the vegetables destroys these enzymes.

I made certain I was not buying any GMO garbage and instead bought fresh vegetables almost all the time. If you simply cannot find fresh vegetables then frozen is the next best thing. As mentioned earlier, canned vegetables were always my last choice. Canned vegetables generally have the vitamins, minerals, antioxidants and phytonutrients boiled out of them during processing.

According to Dr. Baroody, author of the book "Alkalize or Die," 70% - 80% of the vegetables you consume should be raw, as in a salad. Steam the remaining 20% – 30%.

I kept myself and my mother on this strict diet including uncontaminated protein and fresh vegetables, and not much else, for 3 months. The only place we strayed from the suggestions of Dr. Baroody was in the percentages of raw vegetables. We ate half of our vegetables raw instead of the suggested 70% - 80%. The other half I steamed.

As I mentioned earlier, my mother's teeth were weak so I generally took the harder vegetables, like carrots and broccoli, and steamed them. The softer vegetables I cut up and put in bowls so they were ready for salads.

When choosing fish I always made sure it was not from a fish farm. I think these farms contaminate the meat in the same manner that farmers contaminate beef, pork, chicken and lamb, by giving antibiotics and steroids to the animals and feeding them substandard food.

One positive result from the New Menu was that my mother was thinking clearer, she was sleeping a little better and her mood became more consistent with fewer outbursts and less anger. I also experienced improvements in my overall health eating this same food every day. Adapting to this New Menu is difficult but the benefits I personally experienced made sticking to it more than worth it! Keep in mind that you can have as much of the steamed and raw vegetables and protein as you want.

I constantly hear from people saying they are starving on this diet. This is generally because they are eating a small pile of steamed vegetables and a small salad and only one chicken breast. Why not have a large pile of steamed vegetables and a large salad. If you are hungry enough you may even want 2 chicken breasts.

Even though I did not have emphysema, I knew showing support by eating the same foods my mother was eating was necessary. I did not tell my mother all the details at the beginning. She would remind me that we were out of bread or pudding or something else that she wanted and I would conveniently forget it when I made my trip to the store.

After about a month I started craving salads instead of bread and sweets. I never thought I would actually crave salads and raw vegetables but I did. I even woke up one morning craving a spinach salad.

The transition from forcing this diet to enjoying it took my mother and I about a month. After that we looked forward to the salads instead of choking them down like we did in the beginning. We also looked forward to raw vegetables with Ranch dressing for our snacks.

At the beginning, we would cheat one meal a week and have some bread or some sweets as I mentioned before. After a month or so we started having something closer to the New Menu for our cheating meal. We had a number of healthy snacks that included fresh fruit with plain organic yogurt. The fruit depended on what was available fresh.

Some of our favorite choices were fresh pineapple, blueberries, raspberries or strawberries with the yogurt. Even though these choices are very healthy, they do contain sugar albeit natural sugar. For this reason, these healthy fruit snacks were included only once a week. I realized the more sugar my mother ate, whether it was natural, healthy sugar from fruit, or processed sugar in pudding and cake, the longer it would take for her recovery!

Chapter 3: Meal Suggestions and Examples

I mentioned I used marinades for most of the meats and I always bought a variety of different marinades so we did not have the same taste each time. I would generally have at least one or two bowls in the refrigerator marinating meat for future meals. Coming up with breakfast foods was more difficult than lunch and dinner.

I generally made scrambled eggs the night before so I could quickly microwave them in the morning with very little effort. I would cut up ham or bacon and mix it in the eggs even though these meats are not very healthy. The eggs were too boring otherwise and my mother would complain.

I would occasionally add a half of a banana or some orange slices to her plate even though this added sugar to the meal. I also used the microwave which I know is not the healthiest method of cooking but it was fast and I needed shortcuts so I did not feel so overwhelmed.

I always added seasoning to the meats and the vegetables. If the meat was already marinated that was enough seasoning but if it was not, I would add garlic or paprika or oregano or some other seasoning that would enhance the taste. When stir frying I generally added ground ginger when cooking the meat and the vegetables. Adding seasoning will greatly improve an otherwise boring meal or dish.

I generally used vinaigrette dressings on the salads. Many salad dressings are full of sugar, trans fat and other ingredients that are not very healthy. For this reason I limited the salad dressings I bought to the healthier ones. If my mother requested a certain dressing that was not the healthiest I bought it anyway. I figured she would only use a tablespoon or two so the unhealthy ingredients would not have that much affect on slowing her progress.

Condiments are another area where sugar is very common. I read the ingredients on ketchup and a few others and was very surprised how much sugar, or high fructose corn syrup they actually contained. For this reason I provided these condiments very sparingly.

I noticed that if I marinated hamburgers with mesquite flavoring, the burgers did not require ketchup or mustard. I could mix chopped onions into the hamburger before marinating and then grill the burgers for a tastier and healthier main dish. I made the burgers thick so they did not fit well on a bun so my mother would not request a bun or bread with the burger. My intentions were good even if my methods were a tiny bit dishonest.

Breakfast

Breakfast was the most difficult meal with regards to variety. Breakfast so often includes bread or toast, cereals both cold and hot, pastries and fruit, none of which are included in the New Menu. The following are some of the actual meals I made for my mother and I.

Example 1
Scrambled eggs with diced ham
Coffee with powdered cream

Example 2
Fried eggs with 2 slices of turkey bacon
Sliced tomatoes
Coffee with powdered cream

Example 3
Poached eggs with sliced ham
Coffee with powdered cream

Example 4
Omelet with white onions, tomatoes and green peppers
Sliced tomatoes
Coffee with powdered cream

Example 5
Scrambled eggs with diced ham, white onions and crushed garlic
Coffee with powdered cream

Example 6
Hard-boiled eggs with 1 slice of bacon
Sliced tomatoes
Coffee with powdered cream

Example 7
Scrambled eggs with diced ham and green peppers
Coffee with powdered cream

Example 8
Fried eggs with one slice of bacon
Sliced tomatoes
Coffee with powdered cream

Example 9
Fried eggs
Organic sausage
Coffee with powdered cream

Example 10
Omelet with diced tomatoes, white onions and crushed garlic.
Steamed carrots.
Coffee with powdered cream.

Lunch

The lunches I prepared were often leftovers from dinner. I could microwave the meat and the vegetables that were already cooked and make a salad all in less than 5 minutes. For this reason there are not as many lunch examples listed.

Any of the dinner examples will work fine for lunch also. Remember, I am not recommending you follow these foods exactly but rather make your own meals with foods you enjoy.

Example 1
Fresh tomato stuffed with tuna salad, turkey salad or chicken salad
Romaine salad with white onions, zucchini squash and red peppers
Balsamic vinaigrette dressing

Example 2
Soft chicken tacos
Refried beans
Romaine salad with cherry tomatoes and white onions
Balsamic vinaigrette dressing

Example 3
Sliced ham with sliced, fresh pineapple
Sliced tomatoes
Romaine salad with cherry tomatoes and white onions
Balsamic vinaigrette dressing

Example 4
Chicken soup with carrots, white onions and garlic
Sliced tomatoes
Romaine salad with cherry tomatoes, yellow squash and white onions
Balsamic vinaigrette dressing

Example 5
Chef's salad with cubed chicken
Steamed, unpeeled carrots with crushed garlic

Example 6
Ham salad rolled up in Romaine lettuce leaves
Sliced tomatoes
Steamed green beans

Example 7
Chicken salad with sliced tomatoes
Romaine salad with cherry tomatoes and white onions
Balsamic vinaigrette dressing

Example 8
Grilled hamburgers with brown gravy and white onions
Sliced tomatoes
Steamed, fresh green beans
Romaine salad with cherry tomatoes, yellow peppers and zucchini squash
Balsamic vinaigrette dressing

Example 9
Baked, marinated pork steaks with crushed garlic
Steamed fresh green beans
Romaine salad with cherry tomatoes and white onions
Balsamic vinaigrette dressing

Example 10
Tomatoes stuffed with green salad
Steamed asparagus
Romaine salad with cherry tomatoes and white onions
Balsamic vinaigrette dressing

Dinner

Dinner always began with beef, chicken, pork or fish marinated for 24-48 hours and then either baked, grilled or stir fried. If I did not have something marinating I used zesty Italian dressing on chicken breasts on the grill. The dressing made the chicken breasts moist and flavorful.

I used barbecue sauce sometimes even though it is not allowed on the New Menu because of the sugar content. Brushing a little barbecue sauce on the chicken breasts while they grilled created another new taste for a main dish.

The following are some actual meals my mom and I ate during this time:

Example 1
Mesquite marinated hamburgers, grilled
Steamed unpeeled fresh carrots
Romaine salad with green and red peppers, white onions, zucchini squash and summer squash
Balsamic vinaigrette dressing

Example 2
Herb and garlic marinated fish fillets (frozen Pollack) baked at 300 for 30 minutes
Steamed broccoli
Romaine salad with white onions, cherry tomatoes and zucchini squash
Balsamic vinaigrette dressing

Example 3
Southwestern marinated, grilled chicken with fresh lime squeezed on chicken during the last minute of cooking
Steamed fresh green beans with crushed garlic
Sliced tomatoes
Romaine salad with white onions, red, yellow and orange peppers, red onions and cherry tomatoes
Balsamic vinaigrette dressing

Example 4
Garlic and chive marinated pork steaks, baked
Steamed fresh peas and carrots with crushed garlic
Spinach salad with hard-boiled egg, ham and white onions
Balsamic vinaigrette dressing

Example 5
Beef shoulder roast cooked with a package of onion soup in a baking bag
Steamed carrots and green beans with crushed garlic
Sliced tomatoes
Spinach and Romaine lettuce salad with white onions, yellow peppers and cherry tomatoes
Balsamic vinaigrette dressing

Example 6
Teriyaki and ginger marinated chicken strips stir-fried in olive oil (Remember, use coconut oil instead.)
Zucchini squash, summer squash and white onions stir-fried in teriyaki and ginger
Romaine salad with strawberries, cherry tomatoes and white onions with raspberry walnut vinaigrette dressing

Example 7
Beef stew using leftover beef shoulder roast, carrots, green beans, white onions and tomatoes
Steamed Brussels sprouts with crushed garlic
Romaine salad with white onions and cherry tomatoes
Balsamic vinaigrette dressing

Example 8
Homemade chicken soup with vegetable leftovers and dry chicken gravy mix
Spinach salad with cherry tomatoes, white onions and hard-boiled egg
Balsamic vinaigrette dressing

Example 9
Mesquite marinated chicken breasts, grilled
Steamed snow peas and white onions with crushed garlic
Romaine and spinach salad with white onions, zucchini squash and cubed tomatoes
Balsamic vinaigrette dressing

Example 10
Grilled hamburgers mixed with chopped fresh white onions and crushed garlic
Steamed unpeeled carrots with crushed garlic
Spinach salad with cubed Roma tomatoes and zucchini squash
Balsamic vinaigrette dressing

Example 11
Stir-fried, teriyaki marinated beef strips
Red, orange, yellow peppers and white onions stir-fried in ginger
Spinach salad with cherry tomatoes, zucchini and yellow squash
Balsamic vinaigrette dressing
I glass of tomato juice

Example 12
Homemade meatballs with marinara sauce ("No pasta" Italian dish)
Steamed green beans and unpeeled carrots with crush garlic
Romaine salad with cherry tomatoes and white onions
Zesty Italian dressing

Example 13
Three cheese tortellini's with marinara sauce
Fresh ground parmesan cheese
Steamed fresh snow peas with crushed garlic
Spinach salad with cherry tomatoes, zucchini and yellow squash and orange peppers
Balsamic vinaigrette dressing

Example 14
Grilled hamburgers baked in oven with brown gravy and white onions
Steamed fresh green beans and unpeeled carrots with crushed garlic
Romaine salad with cherry tomatoes, white onions and yellow squash
Balsamic vinaigrette dressing

Example 15
Chicken breasts baked with chicken gravy, carrots, white onions and crushed garlic
Steamed green beans with crushed garlic
Sliced tomatoes
Romaine salad with cherry tomatoes, zucchini and yellow squash
Balsamic vinaigrette dressing

Example 16
Grilled lime cilantro chicken breasts
Steamed fresh peas and unpeeled carrots with crushed garlic
Romaine salad with white onions, cherry tomatoes and orange peppers
Balsamic vinaigrette dressing

Example 17
Grilled sirloin steak strips
Steamed green beans with crushed garlic
Sliced tomatoes
Romaine salad with cherry tomatoes and white onions
Balsamic vinaigrette dressing

Example 18
Herb and spice marinated tilapia fish baked at 3000 F for 30 minutes
Steamed red cabbage and white onions with crushed garlic
Romaine salad with cherry tomatoes and white onions
Balsamic vinaigrette dressing

Example 19
Stir-fried chicken strips marinated in ginger and garlic
Stir-fried white onions, red peppers, green peppers and red cabbage
Romaine salad with cherry tomatoes and zucchini squash
Balsamic vinaigrette dressing

Example 20
Grilled pork chops with zesty Italian dressing applied during grilling
Grilled white onions and red peppers with butter and crushed garlic
Spinach salad with cherry tomatoes and yellow squash
Balsamic vinaigrette dressing

Example 21
Homemade chili
Steamed unpeeled carrots with crushed garlic
Spinach salad with hard-boiled eggs and cherry tomatoes
Balsamic vinaigrette dressing

Example 22
Grilled, butterflied organic (no steroids, no antibiotics) Italian sausage
Marinara sauce
Spinach salad with white onions and cherry tomatoes
Balsamic vinaigrette dressing

Example 23
Homemade tacos with fresh diced tomatoes, white onions and grated cheddar cheese
Steamed, unpeeled carrots

Example 24
Baked turkey with gravy
Steamed fresh green beans
Sliced tomatoes
Romaine salad with red peppers, white onions, zucchini and yellow squash

Example 25
Marinated, baked chicken strips
Steamed carrots and white onions with crushed garlic
Romaine salad with cherry tomatoes and white onions
Balsamic vinaigrette dressing

Example 26
Mesquite marinated, grilled sirloin steak strips
Steamed Brussels sprouts with crushed garlic
Spinach salad with hard-boiled eggs, white onions and cherry tomatoes
Balsamic vinaigrette dressing

Example 27
Baked marinated chicken breasts
Steamed asparagus
Romaine salad with red onions and red cabbage
Balsamic vinaigrette dressing

Example 28
Baked, marinated turkey breast with carrots and white onions
Steamed green beans with crushed garlic
Romaine salad with cherry tomatoes and yellow peppers
Balsamic vinaigrette dressing

Example 29
Baked, marinated pork roast with fresh sweet potatoes
Steamed unpeeled carrots and white onions
Romaine salad with cherry tomatoes, yellow and zucchini squash
Raspberry, walnut vinaigrette dressing

Example 30
Baked ham with carrots and white onions
Sliced tomatoes
Steamed green beans
Romaine salad with red peppers, red onions and zucchini squash
Balsamic vinaigrette dressing

Example 31
Homemade meatloaf using Italian bread crumbs (this is a New Menu violation but I used a small amount of bread crumbs anyway.)
Steamed green beans and white onions with crushed garlic
Romaine salad with cherry tomatoes, yellow and orange peppers and red cabbage
Balsamic vinaigrette dressing

Snacks

As I mentioned earlier, this new menu does not offer much in the way of snacks. One snack that my mom really likes is fresh blueberries and plain, organic yogurt. I don't mean vanilla flavored yogurt, I mean the plain yogurt that almost tastes like sour cream. I made this quick snack for my mother and much to my surprise she loved it. Even though fresh blueberries are extremely healthy, the sugar is a no-no on this diet so we only did this occasionally.

My mother and I strictly adhered to the New Menu almost all of the time once we transitioned to it. Sometimes we just could not hang on for another meal and needed something that was not allowed. We would cheat a little and then get right back to the New Menu. I realized it would have been better if we had stayed on the New Menu for three months before cheating. My mom and I did our best and when we just could not stand it any longer, we cheated.

A snack that I liked was almonds. For some people, like my mother, almonds are too hard to chew. If you have similar problems with your teeth, soak the almonds overnight in some distilled or filtered water. If you don't have distilled or filtered water you can use tap but I recommend not using tap water for any consumption unless you do not have other options.

We ate almonds, cashews, walnuts and pecans for snacks on a regular basis. We stayed away from peanuts. Believe it or not, the skin on the peanut and the shell are easily and commonly contaminated with fungi such as mold so I did not include them. Pistachios have the same problem so I did not include them in our snacks either.

At this stage, I wasn't sure what pathogen was proliferating in my mother's lungs but I was pretty convinced that it was there and that it had caused the disease progression even though the doctors disagreed with me.

The reason was that once I started treating her emphysema and COPD as if it were a pathogen she began improving!

My thought was, *"If it walks like a duck and it quacks like a duck, it's a duck!"*

Prior to that, we had followed all the doctors orders which had not produced ONE single improvement in two and a half years!

Another option for a tasty, healthy snack is raw vegetables with a little dip. We used Ranch dressing for the dip and even though it is not really on the New Menu we used such a small amount that I allowed it anyway.

Because of the trouble my mother had with her teeth, I prepared softer vegetables for our snacks like zucchini and yellow squash cut into strips. I would not use them now because they are commonly GMO in fact they are one of the top 8 foods that are likely GMO.

This makes an excellent snack that does not require any preparation since I used vegetables I already had cut up for stir fry. I have found that these vegetables are available at the Organic Farmer's Market so when I want them I buy them there but not at the grocery where GMO is getting more and more common.

Salads make excellent snacks and are very healthy as you probably know. I heard somewhere that you can change a habit in 30 days. Within 30 days of eating salads twice every day my mother and I began craving the raw vegetables that we had to choke down at the beginning. Within a few months, our first choice for a snack was a big salad.

Conclusion

I was amazed that after only two weeks on the strict diet my mother was already improving! I couldn't believe the doctors with all their training did not even suggest this diet that was already making a huge difference in my mother's condition.

They did not even seem interested in questioning the "canned" sounding rhetoric they had been taught by the pharmaceutical industry. Let's face it, doctors are among the most intelligent people in modern society. I couldn't believe they went along with these "medical protocols" and the treatments that they dictated even though these treatments were not working and they knew it!

They called the disease progression of COPD a mystery yet it is obvious that something is growing or proliferating in the lungs of smokers and ex-smokers! Otherwise, why would their COPD worsen for years, even decades after they quit smoking? Even people exposed to second-hand smoke are at risk. It was unfathomable to me that they did not go through the simple process of elimination that I had gone through and realized the only logical, possible cause of this disease must be a pathogen of some sort proliferating in the lungs put there by smoking or breathing second-hand smoke!

This disease was not cancer or it would have been detected as cancer through blood tests and other diagnostics. It was not bacterial or the repeated prescriptions for antibiotics would have killed it. That only leaves viral and fungal. If it were viral this also would have been detected by a blood test. I do however, believe that an "opportunistic fungi" is causing the progression of COPD.

Opportunistic fungi invade the body after the body's probiotics are killed off by antibiotics. Some, like Candida albicans, reside in the body and are kept in check by our probiotics. Once we kill our probiotics with antibiotics a dysbiosis occurs allowing the overgrowth of Candida albicans.

Antibiotics weaken the body's immune response by killing our probiotics which make up 70% - 80% of our immune system. Opportunistic fungi emulate human cells and often go undetected by the body's immune system. As a result the fungal colonies proliferate very slowly. Once they are in the bloodstream they can invade any organ they wish.

Their proliferation can occur over many decades. Most of us know someone who quit smoking and was diagnosed many years, sometimes even decades later with COPD and emphysema. I believe this is due to this slowly proliferating opportunistic fungi.

The bottom line is that I do not believe the progression of COPD is a mystery at all. I definitely believe that if I had relied on the prescribed medications and nebulizer treatments my mother would have died in 2006 from emphysema and COPD.

Once I realized the drugs were only masking symptoms I stopped relying on them for anything else. The pharmaceutical companies that developed these drugs claim they slow the progress of COPD but after watching my mother deteriorate while using them I began thinking some may actually accelerate the disease progression!

I sincerely hope and pray that you will take this disease seriously and realize great success with this diet as my mother and more than 7800 others in 27 different countries already have! I do not believe the medical and pharmaceutical industries will ever embrace these alternative treatments because they work and they do not help sell expensive drugs.

Take a Look at the Difference!

September 2007

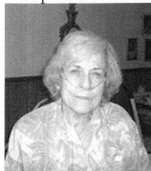

December 2008

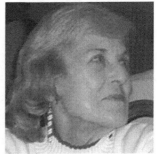

This is my mother in September 2007 in the early stages of recovery from emphysema and COPD.

This is my mother in December 2008 after her complete recovery from emphysema and COPD. Notice there is no longer an oxygen cannula in her nose and she is finally smiling again. Thank God!

About the Author

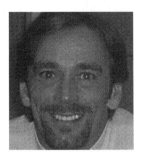

W. Greg Miller worked in the civil engineering field for more than 10 years after receiving his engineering degree. His father was an engineer and they worked together for a number of years inspecting, rating and designing bridges.

When his father passed away, Greg moved into the sales and marketing field. After progressing through the ranks he eventually landed a position as a Regional Manager for a software company running a 5 state area. From there Mr. Miller advanced to a position as the National Marketing Director for a medical software company directing all marketing operations for three offices across the country.

Mr. Miller eventually left that company starting his own software company developing and marketing his own software. While working diligently on marketing these new software programs his mother became ill with emphysema and COPD. Mr. Miller began researching the disease finding all the bad news from the medical and pharmaceutical industries. As his mother's condition deteriorated he eventually moved in and took care of her.

The book, *"How I Reversed My Mom's Emphysema"* is a detailed account of the years that followed, detailing his mother's deterioration to End Stage Emphysema and her eventual and complete recovery!

Since the release of the first edition some 5 years ago, more than 7800 people in 27 different countries have benefited using the protocols and alternative treatments that Mr. Miller used in helping his mother completely recover from emphysema and COPD!

Want the Whole Story Now?!

All of the alternative treatments that were instrumental in reversing his mother's emphysema and COPD were already being used by doctors and researchers working on curing other diseases.

These included Dr. Kenneth Hunter, a Microbiologist and Cancer Researcher at the University of Nevada School of Medicine, Fred Pescatore, M.D., a practicing physician in New York City, Dr. Baroody with his alkalizing principles and Dr. Green, a Naturopath who successfully kept his father alive for 16 years using alternative treatments.

Decide to eliminate all the foods that are not allowed on the diet over the next week and then look for subtle, yet permanent, improvements beginning in the next 2 weeks.

Want the entire story and the book NOW?

Visit our web site.

GET STARTED TODAY!!

www.Emphysema-Treatments.com

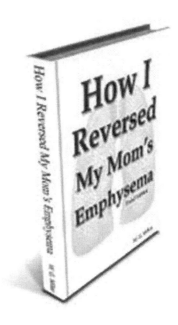

COPD FOCUS GROUPS

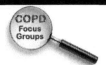

COPD Focus Groups are private groups that assist participants as they proceed through each step and protocol covered in the book from the beginning all the way to complete recovery!

- These groups are only for those serious about recovery that wish to be on the fast track!
- Group size is limited to 10 participants and fill up fast!
- Signup closes at the end of each month.

For information on our NEW - COPD Focus Groups, send me an email to my personal email:

Gmiller5227@yahoo.com

Reverse Emphysema Self Test

SECTION 1: HISTORY

1. Have you taken tetracyclines (Sumycin®, Panmycin®, Vibramycin®, Minocen®, etc.) or other antibiotics for acne for 1 month (or longer)?
Enter 35 for Yes, 0 for No

2. Have you, at any time in your life, taken other "broad spectrum" antibiotics for respiratory, urinary or other infections (for 2 months or longer, or in shorter courses 4 or more times in a 1-year period)?
Enter 35 for Yes, 0 for No

3. Have you taken a broad spectrum antibiotic drug — even a single course?
Enter 6 for Yes, 0 for No

4. Have you, at any time in your life, been bothered by persistent prostatis,
vaginitis or other problems affecting your reproductive organs?
Enter 25 for Yes, 0 for No

5. Have you been pregnant? (enter only 1 answer)
*2 or more times? Enter 5 for Yes, 0 for No
*1 time? Enter 3 for Yes, 0 for No

6. Have you taken birth control pills? (enter only 1 answer)
*For more than 2 years? Enter 15 for Yes, 0 for No
*For 6 months to 2 years? Enter 8 for Yes, 0 for No

7. Have you taken prednisone, Decadron® or other cortisone-type drugs?
(enter only 1 answer)
*For more than 2 weeks? Enter 15 for Yes, 0 for No
*For 2 weeks or less? Enter 6 for Yes, 0 for No

8. Does exposure to perfumes, insecticides, fabric shop odors or other chemicals provoke? (enter only 1 answer)
*Moderate to severe symptoms? Enter 20 for Yes, 0 for No
*Mild symptoms? Enter 5 for Yes, 0 for No

9. Are your symptoms worse on damp, muggy days or in moldy places?
Enter 20 for Yes, 0 for No

10. Have you had athlete's foot, ring worm, "jock itch" or other chronic fungal infections of the skin or nails? Have such infections been,
(enter only 1 answer)
*Severe or persistent? Enter 20 for Yes, 0 for No
*Mild to moderate? Enter 10 for Yes, 0 for No

11. Do you crave sugar or sugar containing foods like desserts and candy?
Enter 10 for Yes, 0 for No

12. Do you crave breads, rolls, muffins or any other grains or foods made from grains? Enter 10 for Yes, 0 for No

13. Do you crave alcoholic beverages including beer or wine?
Enter 10 for Yes, 0 for No

14. Does tobacco smoke really bother you?
Enter 10 for Yes, 0 for No

Enter your responses to the questions in Section 1 below:

1. ____
2. ____
3. ____
4. ____
5. ____
6. ____
7. ____
8. ____
9. ____
10. ____
11. ____
12. ____
13. ____
14. ____

SECTION 1 TOTAL _____

SECTION 2: MAJOR SYMPTOMS

Instructions:
For each symptom that is present, record the appropriate score.
*Record a "0" if a symptom does not apply to you.
*Record a "3" if a symptom is occasional or mild.
*Record a "6" if a symptom is frequent and/or moderately severe.
*Record a "9" if a symptom is severe and/or disabling.

1. Fatigue or lethargy
2. Feeling of being "drained"
3. Poor memory
4. Feeling "spacey" or "unreal"
5. Inability to make decisions
6. Numbness, burning or tingling
7. Insomnia
8. Muscle aches
9. Muscle weakness or paralysis
10. Pain and/or swelling in joints
11. Abdominal pain
12. Constipation
13. Diarrhea
14. Bloating, belching or intestinal gas
15. Troublesome vaginal burning, itching or discharge
16. Prostatitis
17. Impotence
18. Loss of sexual desire or feeling
19. Endometriosis or infertility
20. Cramps and/or other menstrual irregularities
21. Premenstrual tension
22. Attacks of anxiety or crying
23. Cold hands or feet and/or chilliness
24. Shaking or irritable when hungry

Enter your responses to the questions in Section 2 below:

1. _____
2. _____
3. _____
4. _____
5. _____
6. _____
7. _____
8. _____
9. _____
10. _____
11. _____
12. _____
13. _____
14. _____
15. _____
16. _____
17. _____
18. _____
19. _____
20. _____
21. _____
22. _____
23. _____
24. _____

SECTION 2 TOTAL _____

SECTION 3: ADDITIONAL SYMPTOMS

Instructions:

While symptoms in this section commonly occur in patients with illnesses having a fungal component, they also occur commonly in patients who don't. This section acts to reaffirm the results from the first two sections.

For each symptom that is present, record the appropriate score.

Enter a "1" if a symptom is occasional or mild.
Enter a "2" if a symptom is frequent and/or moderately severe.
Enter a "3" if a symptom is severe and/or disabling.

1. Drowsiness
2. Irritability or jitteriness
3. Lack of Coordination
4. Inability to concentrate
5. Frequent mood swings
6. Headaches
7. Dizziness/loss of balance
8. Pressure above ears...feeling of head swelling
9. Tendency to bruise easily
10. Chronic rashes or itching
11. Psoriasis or recurrent hives
12. Indigestion or heartburn
13. Food sensitivity or intolerance
14. Mucus in stools
15. Rectal itching
16. Dry mouth or throat
17. Rash or blister in mouth
18. Bad breath
19. Foot, hair or body odor not relieved by washing

20. Nasal congestion or post nasal drip
21. Nasal itching
22. Sore throat
23. Laryngitis, loss of voice
24. Cough or recurrent bronchitis
25. Pain or tightness in chest
26. Wheezing or shortness of breath
27. Urinary frequency, urgency, or incontinence
28. Burning on urination
29. Spots in front of eyes or erratic vision
30. Burning or tearing of eyes
31. Recurrent infections or fluid in ears
32. Ear pain or deafness

Enter your responses to Section 3 below:

1. _____
2. _____
3. _____
4. _____
5. _____
6. _____
7. _____
8. _____
9. _____
10. _____
11. _____
12. _____
13. _____
14. _____
15. _____
16. _____
17. _____
18. _____
19. _____
20. _____
21. _____
22. _____
23. _____
24. _____
25. _____
26. _____
27. _____
28. _____
29. _____
30. _____
31. _____
32. _____

SECTION 3 TOTAL _____

Total Your Score

Simply add your scores from Section 1, 2, and 3 for your total score then compare your score with the "Understanding Your Score" section below.

Section 1 Score _____

Section 2 Score _____

Section 3 Score _____

TOTAL SCORE _____

Understanding Your Score

Your Total Score will provide a strong indication of whether you will benefit from the information in the book, "How I Reversed My Mom's Emphysema." Scores in women will run higher since 7 items in the questionnaire apply exclusively to women, while only 2 apply exclusively to men.

Women: 180 or more
Men: 140 or more
It is extremely likely you would benefit from the information in the book.

Women: 120 or more
Men: 90 or more
It is probable you would benefit from the information in the book.

Women: 60 or more
Men: 40 or more
It is quite possible you would benefit from the information in the book.

Women: less than 60
Men: Less than 40   Does not necessarily mean that you would not benefit from the information in the book, it just means it was not evident from the results of this test.

"When I did this test for my mother she scored a 264!"

She recovered 17 months later by following the protocols in the book!

DON'T DELAY!

GET YOUR COPY TODAY!

VISIT OUR WEB SITE!

www.Emphysema-Treatments.com

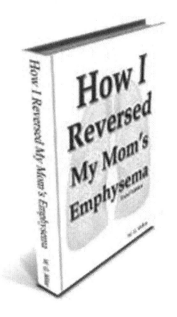

"This could be the best decision you ever make!"

Made in the USA
Middletown, DE
22 June 2017